The Good Enema

By
J G Knox

LTL Publishing
PO Box 65130
Vancouver, WA 98665
United States
1-360-690-0842

©

Copyright 2009

by
J.G. Knox
All Rights Reserved

No part of this book may be reproduced by any mechanical, photographic or electronic process, or in the form of phonographic recording, nor may it be stored in a retrieval system, transmitted, translated into another language, or otherwise copied for public or private use, except brief passages quoted for purposes of review, without the written permission of the author.

ISBN 978-0-9842381-9-4

Table of Contents

Prologue 1

My Turn 3

Her Turn 17

Veterans 35

Dedication

This story is dedicated to the Good Enema, a treatment older than written language, used throughout history to treat hundreds of medical conditions, and currently out of fashion.

Forward

"And now abideth faith, hope, and charity, these three: but the greatest of these is charity." In the Bible, charity is love. The thirteenth chapter of First Corinthians, the central passage defining Christianity, ends with this verse. Yet in modern corporate culture, money matters: hope, faith, and love don't. The Bible goes to the essence of this, not forgetting profit, but properly placing it in relationship to love. It says: "The love of money is the root of all evil." I Timothy 6:10. Not money itself, but the love of it.

Money is a tool. Love is the purpose, not a tool. When the accumulation of money is the purpose of every act, and of every service, then the purpose of life is missed. It isn't just Christianity that makes love the key test of life: it's all the major religions. All deplore the making of money a supreme goal. All equate love with God.

When doctors made house calls, knew their patients, when they based their lives on serving patients, and were paid in the cries of babies born, in heart-felt thanks, and in bushel baskets of beans, corn, and vegetables; enemas were common.

The use of the enema grew to an art and science in a different time. A time when the skills and practice of every knowledgeable nurse and doctor was based on human, not corporate, values: on doing what was best for patients, not best for corporations.

Good doctors, of that era, knew that the taking and holding of a large warm enema warmed the core of the body, stimulated the immune system, and helped the patient's own body fight off colds, flu, and other systemic infections. They knew that the taking and expelling of a good enema helped a woman in labor to relax and get into the rhythm of bearing down to have her baby, with a shorter labor and less pain. They knew that the giving of a good enema was the first thing to be done in the treatment and cure of many conditions. They also knew that the giving of good enemas was not profitable. No doctor or nurse ever got rich giving enemas. Enemas are a way to help people, not make money. It was a different time.

Human motivation doesn't change. Doctors and nurses go into health care to serve others. The essence of good medicine, of any system of healing, is helping the patient. If that love of others is not the center of motivation, the system fails. Health care isn't about money. Money is no more an agent of healing than the use of any other tool. It shouldn't be about the love of money, but is.

The enema, one of the most common treatments in all branches of health care, began to be systematically purged from hospitals, doctor's offices, and home health care when corporations took over: when profit became the only criteria of success in American health care. Corporations never understand hope, faith, and love; but they understand money. They recognize and practice one principle: making profit!

Neither enemas, nor love, can compete in a system where the only motivation allowed to be judged is making profit. Enemas are time consuming, potentially messy, and don't generate money back to corporate headquarters.

The elimination of enemas, and any other form of care, which does nothing to support the supreme goal of corporations, making money, has permeated modern

American health care, and is sinking it. America has the most profitable health-care system in the world. Americans pay more for health care than any other country. According to the Organization for Economic Co-ordination and Development (OECD), in America we paid $7,290 per person for health care in 2007. The second highest, Norway, paid $4,763. Other countries trailing far behind in cost provided better health care to their citizens. In the 2000 assessment of the World Health Organization, America was thirty-seventh among nations in the over-all quality of health care delivered to its people, just behind Costa Rica. American health quality is now ranked lower than it was in 2000, but does lead the world in pharmaceutical development and many areas of medical research. And we are a health-care destination for the wealthy of the world, who are willing to spend hundreds of thousands of dollars, out of pocket, for health-care procedures that average Americans cannot afford.

It's not the doctors, nurses, or workers, nor science, that is the driving force behind this decline. The design and function of corporations is to make money, and their power has grown to such a level than no person, or group of people within the corporate system, can inject human values. We are all swept up in this. The values of hope, faith, and love are lost: the value of serving patients is lost.

Serving the people is not even being mentioned in the current battle over health care reform in America. The prime topic of discussion is how to pay for it, how to keep the insurance companies in control, and how to keep profit as the main motivator driving American health care. The reality is---unless human values regain control, unless love again becomes part of the motivation of providing health care, our future is dark, unhealthful, and corporate profits will evaporate as our nation implodes.

The enema, a most unprofitable treatment, is gone from our system of corporate health care, yet does not go away. People discover its usefulness, its benefits to health. But, if knowledge of how to use enemas, how they feel, and their benefits in health care can be suppressed, patients may forget, doctors and nurses may forget, and corporate profit alone may continue to rule our health care system.

But can a system driven by profit only continue to make money when the needs of patients are ignored? Our system is failing not because profit is wrong. It's not. What's wrong is loving it, making it the purpose, not just a tool. Love is something between patients and health-care providers, parents and children, between people. Love is the supreme value. Without it, life is meaningless.

All financial tools, including corporations, are tools. They are not people, and must never have the rights of people. Used as tools, relegated to their proper position in the rule of law and personal action, all tools have their place and use. When paper creations become gods, when they become regarded as living entities, when they destroy life to enhance paper profits, when humans submit to the rule of lifeless corporations, death rules. Health care is not about death; it's about life.

The Bible, I Corinthians 13:3, says: "And though I bestow all my goods and feed the poor, and though I give my body to be burned, and have not charity, it profiteth me nothing." Without love, without life, profit cannot long exist. Short-term profits can be recorded on dead paper ledgers, feeding off the dead corpses of civilizations, but without life, profit cannot continue.

This book, and the others I write, are not dedicated to profit, but to love. The enema is a good treatment. For many thousands of years, enemas have been given as described in this book. The feelings, the love, and the uses of enemas are what *The Good Enema* is about, what this part of health care was like before the rule of corporate medicine. It is our goal to share love, to share knowledge, and to share the art of caring for others and ourselves. Our motivation is to bring health to patients, and to do this in ways that are proven, and work.

We have a web site, http://www.lifeknox.com, giving some conditions treated by enemas: candida, irritable bowel syndrome, constipation, colds & flu, preparation for childbirth, etc., and an article on how to give an enema, which will be part of a new publication on how and why to give enemas.

Good enemas will return to health care. Helping our children, friends, wives and husbands, mothers and fathers, patients, people who trust us with their care, will be based on love again. "And now abideth faith, hope, and love, these three: but the greatest of these is love," I Corinthians 13:13. All other things will pass away.

Read, *The Good Enema* with love.

J. G. Knox, September 2009

Prologue

"I'm going to give you a good enema," has anyone said that to you; have you heard it, not looking up, not able to face the eyes behind the voice; knowing that in minutes you will be naked, a nozzle in your bottom, a bulging bag of water hanging over you; knowing that your rectum will pulsate with waves of water until you're full, until you can't take any more, until quivering you beg her to stop, to let you go to the bathroom; knowing that after she removes the nozzle, covers your nakedness with sheets and blankets, that you will lie holding the enema within you, a wet and ferocious thing moving, living, powered by the contractions of your own colon, clawing at your anus to get out, until she thinks it's time, until she thinks the enema has accomplished its purpose; knowing that you are about to experience one of the most embarrassing, most psychologically challenging and most intimate of medical procedures: have you been given a good enema?

I have.

My Turn

8:00PM, May 10, 1945, visiting hours over, leisurely sauntering down the hall, zipping his flight jacket, the one with the United States Army Air Corps insignias on it, George, a B-25 navigator, came home, safe, well. Why didn't he stay home, keep being principal at Madison High School? He could have gotten a deferment. He didn't. Why didn't he tell me he fell out of a plane doing a routine inspection, dislocated his shoulder, and was reassigned to administrative staff? I thought he was flying, too old to be flying---so did his commander. The general needed a man who was used to managing young men. Most of his flyers, being the age of my husband's former high school students, he was more useful on the ground than in the air.

I told George that and could have told the general that two years earlier.

"A military secret," George said, not wanting to admit he was too old to compete with the younger men in his unit.

I worried the entire time my husband was gone. Nine other men in the Air Corps from the West Side died. Cars stopped delivering telegrams to their wives or mothers. Every time the door bell rang, a car pulled up or stopped on the street in front of our house, I got a knot in my stomach, got diarrhea. Shouldn't the diarrhea have gotten better when he came home? It got worse, worse than it was the day he got his orders for overseas. Now, he worried about me, took me to the doctor. At thirty-four, was I too old to be a navigator's wife?

In the hall the nurse said, "Goodnight, Colonel."

He said, "Goodnight."

The diminutive nurse poked her head into my room.

I smile at her, not knowing her intentions, not knowing what she was going to do to me. A patient in a hospital bed, an object, a slab of flesh assigned to room 4-A was it her turn to probe me, stick me, or feed me some pill? What would she say? I waited.

She spoke.

"Mrs. Johnson?" She confirmed my identity, making sure I was the right slab of flesh.

I nodded.

"I'm going to give you a good enema," she said.

My roommate, a sixteen year old girl, dropping her magazine, letting it slide off her lap, red pages fluttering to the floor, the noise and the colorful motion drew my attention to her. Staring at me, her mouth open, she showed the emotions, the panic, I felt.

My nurse's statement turned my ears pink. My roommate's reaction turned my face red. A good enema, a common hospital procedure, was routine to the nurse, out of the ordinary for me, and a lightning bolt on a dark night for my roommate.

The girl's strong reaction was the reaction of one young, unpracticed at hiding emotions, and knowing intimately the possibilities of a good enema. My reaction was one of a grown woman, able to hide emotions, unable to deal with my own childhood, my own insecurity of losing control of my bowels: unable to forget myself as a four year old girl messing my Easter dress in Sunday school, being an embarrassment to my mother, knowing intimately the meaning of failing to hold in the contents of my colon.

"I'm going to give you a good enema," her mother said seven weeks before, only it wasn't to someone else her mother was speaking. It was to her.

Now I was going to have a good enema. The girl looked at me, a look of recognition, of empathy, of disbelief that this could happen to a grown up, like me.

The nurse said, "I want you to go to the bathroom, urinate, try to have a BM, and I'll be back to give you your enema in twenty minutes.

The staring teenager made me nervous. I slipped off my bed, my panties and pajama bottoms sliding over the sheets. The next time I slid off my bed there would be no panties. I would be in a hurry. I smiled a nervous smile at the teen. She kept looking, didn't smile.

Looking at the nurse, the girl said, "I have a headache. Can I have an aspirin?"

The nurse said, "Of course, Ellen," and went to get her one.

I went to the toilet.

In the toilet, I could urinate, but defecating wasn't possible. Nothing there, why did I need an enema?

Back in my room, I didn't speak. I tried to read my new copy of Look magazine. The girl kept glancing at me. I glanced at her. I knew the routine: two kids, and a barium enema three years ago, nurses had given me enemas before. But, enemas are invasive, embarrassing, and something private. Why, every time this happened, did it have to happen in a semi-private room with an audience: the last time before a barium enema was with an old lady who kept asking, "You all right, honey?", or twelve years before that with another mother-to-be in the next bed? At least in the maternity ward, we took turns having enemas. If we were rich, I would have gotten a private room, wished I had gotten a private room, with no teenage girl in the next bed giving me furtive glances.

Coming back in at twenty minutes on the dot, the nurse carried a treatment tray, a pitcher, a stainless-steel irrigation can, two-liter capacity with a coil of rubber hose and an enema nozzle attached, all uncovered, all exposed for the world to look at, everyone in the hall knowing one of the slabs of flesh in room 4-A was about to have an enema. Did it make me feel better knowing that half a dozen other such trays, and half the nurses and patients on the floor were doing the same thing?

Tray and all, the nurse disappeared into the toilet. Water running, some splashing, the girl and I knew what was happening, kept exchanging glances. The nurse emerged, the pitcher and enema can sitting upright on the tray; the nozzle, not hidden, dangling off the edge. Putting them on my table, the nurse smiled. My roommate's gaze gravitated to the tray, ogling the full enema can, the full pitcher or the enema nozzle, with quick glances toward the nurse, then me.

The nurse laid my bed flat, extended a metal arm at the head of my bed leaving the hook on the end above the middle of the bed, and lifted the enema can to the hook. The girl's mouth was open, her eyes wide and dilated as she watched this. The nurse looped the hose and nozzle over the hook.

Sensing my unease, the nurse pulled the privacy curtain. Gone were penetrating brown eyes watching every move; not gone was the embarrassment heightened by the girl's unwanted attention. In view was the can, the hose, the nozzle, and the nurse's friendly smile. My ears warm and glowing, I couldn't make eye contact with the woman who in seconds would be probing my most private orifice.

She said, "OK, how'd you do in the toilet?"

"I urinated. I'm not constipated. Why do I need an enema?"

"It's not for constipation. The doctor needs you cleaned out, ordered good enemas till clear."

"Oh---" *Did she say enemas?*

"Slip off your pajama bottoms and panties."

I did.

"Lift up."

I did, the nurse slipping a pad under my hips. I pulled the sheet up over my exposed pubic hair, tried to arrange and smooth it making me look more lady like.

The nurse lifted the enema can and hung it on an IV stand a couple of feet above the bed and uncoiled the enema hose. Lowering the bed flat she said, "OK, turn over on your stomach."

I didn't say much. What could I say? Naked from my waist down, being pumped full of water by a stranger, enemas are standard medical practice, but enemas are exposing and inhibiting. Watching my nurse lubricate the nozzle did not lubricate the flow of words. Anything I might have said slipped out of my mind as my panties slipped off my bottom and lay crumpled, silent at my feet. She picked up the edge of the sheet, the sheet I had so carefully covered myself with, and lowered it below my knees, exposing me in the lighted room in a way not even my husband had seen me since he came home. My nurse left no doubt that I was a woman, a female. Can a lady be a lady lying in a lighted room, having her anus probed by a stranger? I was a lady, a prim, proper colonel's lady, wore my hair up, kept my dresses the right length, never swore and never mentioned bowel movements, much less enemas. I was a lady, didn't feel like a lady, felt like a bare A-4 slab of flesh.

"OK," she put her hand around my right hip and pulled it back. "Bend your right knee." She patted my right knee as I brought it up, then just a little bend in my left one. Then nothing, she wasn't touching me.

Looking over my shoulder, I saw her grasping the hose behind the nozzle. I closed my eyes. Her hand was on my buttock, lifting, opening.

"OK, just a little tingle and I'll have the nozzle in."

I barely felt it. My cheeks came together. Then moving my legs slightly, I felt the hose and the nozzle. It was in me.

She said, "Breathe deep and relax."

An almost noiseless click, the hose warmed a path up my leg. The nozzle warmed my anus and a pool of 103 degree Fahrenheit water filled my rectum. She didn't need to ask; the changing temperature of hose in her hand told her. We knew it was going in.

A rhythm: as I breathed in, the vibrating nozzle slowed under the pressure; as I breathed out a relaxing, the vibration in my anus increased as the water coming through the nozzle increased. My eyes closed; I followed the rhythm. A good feeling, a tingling of tender tissue, the enema was feeling good, relaxing, warm, soothing. I relaxed. She rocked my hip.

With my eyes closed, I didn't see my nurse rise on her toes to look into the enema can. Minutes passed. The relaxing rhythm of breathing, surging, vibrating, and taking in water continued unabated. My abdomen inched forward, bulging out with water. A warmth in my gut and a hotness in my bottom---it was a good enema.

Warmth gurgled over my stomach. Tightening, a slow, steady contraction hardened my abdomen. A rumble inside me pressed down. A surge hit my rectum, tried to force its way through my anus. My eyes opened. I squeezed my bottom shut. I held it in. I panted, looked with desperate glances toward my nurse.

"I---I can go now!"

"Breathe deep, it'll ease up." My nurse smiled, rocked my hip.

I looked at her. She rose on her tip toes looking down into the enema can. I breathed deep. She clicked the clamp shut, the vibration stopped.

Water sloshing in my gut, I watched her lift the pitcher and pour the can full again.

"You're doing fine," she said.

She released the clamp. Another full can of enema, Could I hold that much?

The nozzle vibrated. I quivered. A ripple, another wave, another squeezing back, holding on, I needed to go to the bathroom!

She said, "Hold on," a calm, sure "hold on."

She wasn't taking the enema, but giving it, subject to very different emotions, or lack of emotions. She smiled with colorless ears.

My ears once pink with embarrassment, not pale with panick, I said, "I really need to go!"

My roommate cleared her throat. She was listening!

Rubbing my back, not stopping the flow, my nurse kept my enema coming. I breathed short, shallow breaths. Holding more than two quarts, how much enema had I taken? My back tensed.

She clicked the clamp shut.

I exhaled.

The nurse said, "You're doing good. Keep breathing." Rocking my hip at least a minute that time, the nurse smiled.

My urgency eased, passed with a rumble in my abdomen. I smiled.

She said, "Ready?"

I, not answering, looked ahead, heard the clamp unclasp. The enema started again.

Watching me, not asking me, the nurse cut the flow of water off and on, worked me until I thought I would explode, then closed the clamp. With her releasing the clamp, me breathing out, holding the exhalation, moving my legs, then clenching my bottom around the enema hose, we danced. She held the hose, the clamp. I held the nozzle. Three times she opened and closed the clamp. I emptied my lungs and held my breath out, sucking more water up my colon, trying to postpone the filling pressure in my rectum. Breathing in, pushing water back into my rectum, the surge pressed on my anus demanding release. Suppressing the urge, I froze. Outside, I was still as a corpse; inside, I was panicking, running, alive with surges and urges.

My nurse held the clamp, could close the flow of water off with a flick of her thumb. With the small round pipe surrounded by the strongest muscles in my body, what could I do? Squeezing the nozzle with my buttocks and moving my legs, the hard, plastic nozzle did not give, did not stop pouring water into me. As useless as tightening my buttocks to stop a paddling, the enema kept coming.

She had my life in her hand; as surely as, my teacher had the day I was caught smoking under the bleachers. That day I clenched my bottom as the paddle made contact. The paddle kept flowing back and forth until my teacher was ready to stop, until I was crying rivers of tears, until she put the paddle down on the desk, and released it from her hand. I never smoked again. I was never paddled again.

As I was required to lean over the teacher's desk and take it, I stayed on the bed for my nurse and took it. For my teacher, I stood motionless, cried, and danced a jig with my hands on my bottom when it was over.

Working with my teacher with a paddle in her hand, no breaks, a steady rhythm of swats achieving correction, the last spank of the paddle impacted my bottom. The pain ebbed. Learning my lesson, reflecting, I struggled to hold back my tears.

Struggling to hold in my enema was as intense as that paddling, but nothing to learn, no pain, a pleasant good feeling, urgency replacing embarrassment, my buttocks relaxed as the clamp clicked. She gave me a break.

Outside I wasn't crying; I was stoic. Inside, I was doing a jig, dancing around the clamp on the enema hose, dancing to the music the nurse was creating with her bag and pipe. She was playing me as a master plays the bagpipes: bagpipes that can be heard for miles, drawing the lads from the hills for the war, drawing the lasses for the dancing. A nurse with a bag and pipe can coax the bravest lad out of his kilt, the happiest lassie out of her skirt, and make music that smells awful, inspires runs, and is difficult to dance to. Celtic music in my abdomen, I rumbled an abdominal, dour, awful tune.

Tiring, having trouble breathing against the gathering of the clans in my belly, I lulled into the rhythm, the unsustainable rhythm of the pipe, the steady drone of the bag. The warmth of the enema, the flow could keep coming forever, as long as there was water in the can. Not my colon, finite in space, finite in capacity, I was sure my colon was full, wanted the games to end, the pipe to withdraw from my bottom and the bag to be marched away.

My nurse's hand slid around my ilium, pushed on my lower right abdomen, played another organ, one not yet filled.

My nurse said, "It's not full yet; we need your cecum filled and dilated."

The vibration in my anus continued. A wall of contractions surged back and forth, I moved my legs.

I said, "I can't hold anymore!"

She said, "Breathe deep."

The enema continued.

Then another surge, this one above, not pushing, not threatening to spew out of me, went into that area of my right lower abdomen. No pressure below, my nurse rubbed me, closed her eyes felt for my colon.

"OK, that's better," she said.

The enema continued.

Next the pressure came and went in my rectum, increasing crescendos, pressure, relaxing, pressure, relaxing. I held on. I panted, looking back over my shoulder. Would she stop? *Please stop!*

My legs began to quiver. I heard a click. The clamp!

My nurse stopped, said, "You did well."

She held my bottom with one hand, pulled the nozzle out with the other.

"How much enema did you give me?"

"Over three quarts, a good enema" she said.

"Can I go to the bathroom?"

"No, you need to hold it for fifteen minutes."

"Ohhhhh," I said.

"You need to let it work in you, dissolve everything. I'll come back when it's time for you to go. Here let me help you. It'll be better if you lay on your right side, let the water pool on the right to clean your cecum out."

I was moving like an old woman---no, not an old woman, a woman with a full colon. Every motion pressed against the bloated, no longer elastic piping in my abdomen, made the holding the "good enema" harder, made moving around harder.

"Is my cecum the problem?"

"No, just need to fill it," she said. "The cecum's the first part of your colon. A good enema fills the cecum, dissolving everything and washing it down. Otherwise, we have to do more enemas to clear you out."

In position on my right side, she lifted the sheets covering my nudity, straightening the edges, restoring my lady hood.

"Thank you," I said.

I was four-years old again, back in church, sitting in my Sunday school class, feeling powerful urges, holding on. I closed my eyes, saw Momma's smile. This time my mother would be proud of me.

My nurse opened the privacy curtain saying, "I'll be back in 15 minutes."

Earlier her promise of 20 minutes wasn't important. If it were 30, I wouldn't have cared. 15 minutes, squeezing my bottom together holding surges, 15 minutes would be a long time.

Ellen's smile greeted my opening eyes.

She said, "Are you alright?"

"I need to go to the bathroom!"

Ellen said, "My Mom gives me and my brother enemas, sometimes."

I said, "I have a daughter your age---Shannon."

"Do you give her enemas?"

We were going to talk about enemas, a strange topic, a current topic. A surge of water stretched my rectum. I lost my voice, suppressing the surge.

Ellen said, "I think it's important for kids to have enemas."

I said, "Have you talked to other kids about this?"

"No, kids don't talk about enemas, we just need them, and we need our Moms to give them to us."

I said, "Tell me about the enemas your Mom gives you."

Ellen said, "I haven't talked to anybody about it---You don't mind. You want me too---really?"

"I have had some enemas too, never talked about them either. If you want to talk, I'll listen. Holding this enema, I'm not going to be good at talking back, but I'd like to hear what you have to say."

Ellen said, "There's a lot I want to say. Maybe I could just tell you what happened."

Her Turn

"Mom, I don't need an enema!" Ellen said, following her mother to the hallway and watching her retrieving the enema bag and two towels from the hall closet.

Her mother carried the enema; Ellen carried the towels.

"Mom, I don't want an enema!" She said, following her mother into the master bedroom.

"Close the door, Honey," her mother said.

Ellen closed the bedroom door and looked at her mother's bed, neat, with a pale blue quilt-spread embroidered with yellow flowers. Her mother's favorite, made by Ellen's grandmother, her mother didn't even like people sitting on it. An enema on it was out of the question leaking on it was out of the question. Ellen folded the bedspread back off the half of the bed closest to the bathroom and laid the towels neatly on the spot where her hips would go. She fluffed the pillow for her head and looked back at the towels.

Would they be brown stained? Would she run to the toilet leaking, splattering enema water on the tile floor and throw rugs? Not a question the last time she had an enema, it was now.

Her mom had picked her up by herself from school three weeks before. Her brother, David was sick at home, and they stopped by the drug store.

"I got it, Mrs. Black," Mr. Anderson, the druggist said.

Her mom took the flat box, opened it looking at the contents, and handed it to Ellen.

"It's more expensive than the smaller ones." Mr. Anderson named a price.

"Thank you," Her mother said, and paid him.

Ellen was closing the box, hoping none of her classmates saw her mother, or her holding the bag. Even holding the bag in its box was embarrassing. Ellen read the label on the side of the large red bag before getting it securely in the box, Devol, 4 quart capacity; it was a combination hot-water bottle, enema, douche syringe. A curious young mind, Ellen had studied the bag they had at home. A Devol, too, it had the same lettering, but said, Devol, 2 quart capacity. Why a new bag? Why one that held twice as much?

Ellen hurried to the car clutching the syringe close to her chest. She wanted in the car quickly so she could shove it under the dash before anyone saw it. Whether she was carrying it or her mother was, if anyone saw it, the result would be the same. Her mother plus her, plus the enema bag---everyone would assume it was for Ellen, would picture her on her side, bare bottomed taking an enema from this bag. Walking quick, keeping her head down, trying not to attract attention had worked: no one saw her. But, now, at the car, she was stuck standing holding the bag for everyone on the street to see. Her mother stopped chatting with a friend from church, standing by the drug store's front door, in no hurry. Panic. Her mother locked the car; left Ellen holding the bag.

Should she call out for her mother to hurry? That would only attract more attention. Ellen put the box behind her against the car door and leaned on it, trying to cover it with her back. She thought of taking her sweater off and completely covering the box, but that too would attract attention.

A terrible thought rumbled though Ellen's mind, *Was the front of the box, with the nurse on it, the enema bag emblazoned on the corner, framed by her back, visible from the side walk?*

Ellen started to look, and then decided to feel the edge of the box with the hand holding it. The bottom edge came open slightly, while rubbing along her fingers.

She relaxed; the unmarked bottom of the box faced the window. The edge was visible from under the edge of her skirt. It wasn't a perfect solution. Devol combination: hot-water bottle, enema, douche syringe was visible, but the lettering was small enough that it couldn't be read at a distance.

At least, the serious looking nurse staring out on the face of the box couldn't be seen. Everyone knew that nurse, attractive, in uniform, no smile; she was a no-nonsense kind of nurse---the kind that gave good enemas.

Ellen's friend, Halley, noticed it the month before Ellen's Mom bought it. Halley spent three weeks in the hospital with pneumonia that winter. She lay in bed with nothing to do except to keep breathing. Three times a day, till the pneumonia broke, a nurse, like the one on the box, gave her a large warm baking soda enema. She knew enemas, dreamed about having enemas, took a breath and became totally silent anytime anyone mentioned an enema.

They were walking by the drug store; Mr. Anderson had put a display of syringe bags in the front window, one with this nurse on the box behind the bag.

"Look at her," Halley said, bugging her eyes up. "I bet she gives good en---" She stopped; she almost said enema.

Ellen blushed.

Halley turned pale and didn't say anything more.

Halley couldn't even say the word enema; the word frightened her; she almost died. Two other girls, in her pneumonia ward, did die. No penicillin then, no miracle drugs, there was only enemas, bed rest, plasters and hope. Good, warm, baking soda enemas warm the body, hydrate the body, loosen phlegm, and increase immune responses. Did Halley's enemas help her live? Whether they did or not, the association was still there, the coughing, the weakness, and the little girl next to her unable to breathe, unable to stop coughing, turning blue, dying. Halley shivered looking at the bag, remembered the hospital, remembered the enemas and remembered the girl dying. She turned pale, not red.

Halley and Ellen walked down the street in silence for a block before they saw a boy, a good looking boy, a boy in their class, Wilber. Ellen saw him first and started talking about him. Getting her color back, Halley opened up and talked about him. They watched him peddle his bike down the street disappearing around a corner. Nothing more said about the enema syringe. Did either girl forget the "almost conversation," about enemas, or the nurse's face on the enema box?

Looking at the enema bags in a display window was embarrassing; carrying it to the car for her mother would be an ultimate humiliation, if Ellen were seen by Halley or any of her friends. She would turn red. If Halley saw her---did Ellen know how Halley would feel? Would Halley enjoy the embarrassment of her friend, the impending nudity, lack of control or the filling of her bowel, or would she panic inside, think Ellen was sick, worry about her until she saw her at school the next day? Ellen's worries were much earthier.

Why didn't her mother stop gabbing and open the car door.

HURRY MOM! Ellen thought.

Eventually, she came. Ellen dove in the car, crushing the box far under the dash.

"Be careful, Ellen, you'll damage the enema bag," her mother said.

Ellen breathed out a sigh of relief. It was out of sight. She breathed in a new worry. It wasn't a hot-water bottle or a female thing for her mother. It was an enema bag.

"Mom, why do you need a new enema bag? What's wrong with the old one?"

"It doesn't give good enemas anymore. You and David are growing up. You need a bigger bag."

An expiring thought, Ellen gulped, and then remembered, David was sick, not her. She breathed in again.

At home Ellen fiddled with her school books and didn't get out of the car when her mother did. She waited for her mother to unlock the door, and then dashed in the house carrying the offending bag.

David was lounging on the couch under two blankets, asleep, his English book lying on the floor, the radio on, but unheard.

Her mother didn't wake him; slipping upstairs with the enema bag, her mother had plans. David slept easier not knowing those plans. Ellen followed her a few minutes later with the pretext of using the bathroom. The door to her mother's bedroom open, Momma had folded the bedspread back and laid out the towels. Water splashed. Their mother was in the master bathroom assembling and rinsing out the new enema bag.

Ellen said, "You're going to give David an enema?"

"Yes," her mother said.

More relief, complete relief, Ellen was sure the enema wasn't for her. Now she was curious.

She thought, *The new bag gave better enemas*?

Good at keeping important secrets, at least ones that let her spy, when spying was necessary, Ellen had discovered an additional benefit of their heating system. The duct from the furnace ran from to the vent by the bed in her mother's bedroom to the vent in Ellen's room.

Two years earlier David had been in a fight at school. His teacher called and asked to see her mother.

Their 1937 De Soto Coup Sedan, with headlights mounted on the fenders, was parked in front of the school when Ellen came out of class. On their way home, David kept up the pleading of his innocence---well, not actually innocence. As he put it, the other boy needed a whupping.

His mother said, "That makes two of you."

David knew what two meant. He wanted to talk his way out of it. Ellen could see him thinking, trying to come up with a better reason for the fight, for his breaking the school's, and their mom's rules.

A one-sided conversation, their mom said, "He is seven inches shorter than you, David, and you outweigh Billy by more than 70 pounds, and you needed to whup him? That's a beating, not a fight. You have to learn your size, son, not be a bully. You don't fight boys half your size. We're lucky the principal didn't suspend you. Do you have ANYTHING reasonable to say for yourself?"

What is it that robs children of that quick gift of gab, the free flow of unique ideas, reasons that on calm days can bring belly laughs and forgiveness from teachers, principals, and Moms---a spontaneity that evaporates when the mention of whupping, spanking, paddling or other forms of corporal punishment severe enough to bring tears to unrepentant eyes is imminent? David saw in his mind the paddle coming out from under the bed. He felt his bottom reddening. But, as with all humans, he could not remember pain, not the pain of his last paddling, not the pain of the shot in his jaw at the dentist when he had his tooth pulled, nor the pain of breaking his finger during basketball practice. Each pain different, each bad, he taped his finger and was back shooting hoops as soon as it stopped hurting; if he had another tooth pulled he wanted the shot; and he would do anything to avoid or delay this paddling. He sat in the front seat of our car, by Mom, imagining the paddling happening, unable to feel it, numb, dumb; he was unable to speak, unable to visualize another end to this scene. For him, it was a long ride home: six blocks.

Once home, Ellen and her mother got out and went into the house. Opening the door, her mom let Ellen in and looked back at her brother, sitting in the car, his bottom happily sitting on mohair seat covers: the touch mohair better than the touch of leather this time. Their father promised them a new Cadillac---a black one, with leather seats. Before the war, before his restaurant closed after seventy-three percent of the students at the university enlisted, or were drafted and stopped eating there, and before their father enlisted. No Cadillac, no leather seats, no being able to appeal to his father to avoid the paddle. Upstairs waited a strip of leather designed for his seat. He stayed in the car.

Summoning him, Mom said, "Come, David'!

David followed her to her bedroom. His head down, he awaited the touch of leather.

Ellen didn't say a word all the way home---not until dinner. Wanting to avoid any involvement in what was about to happen and Mom's eye, Ellen knew their mother took care of all business at once when it came to paddlings. Ellen didn't think she was in any trouble, but why take a chance? She ducked in her room and planned to stay there reading, or maybe to slip out and play with Halley, if her mom would let her.

Ellen doesn't know why she did, but instead of lying in her bed or reading in her chair, she lay down on the floor. There Ellen discovered acoustics: the science of sound transmission. With her head by the heater vent she could hear every word they were saying as if she were in the same room.

David said, "Mom, I won't do it again."

"Of course you won't, David---or you'll get paddled again. You know the rules, fighting at school means paddling at home, and fighting with a boy half your size means a memorable paddling at home."

Ellen knew, without seeing, what their mother was doing. She was folding the bedspread back. Their mother didn't want any stains on it, including salty tears.

Their mom said, "Lower your pants and lay down."

David, three inches taller than their mother, and heavier, was standing, looking down into her eyes. He wanted to say "no," keep his pants up, not let her paddle him to tears, and defy her, not have the paddling. But, never defying defied their Mother, he was a child, a big child. He did what she ordered. Hands the size few men ever have wrapping around the metal work at the head of his mother's bed, his pants tangling around his knees, he would cry. She would paddle him. He would lower his pants and lay down, but he would be slow about doing it.

No more sounds came out of the vent until the popping of the paddle echoed in Ellen's ears. Three or four pops and David was sobbing.

"I'm sorry, Mom!" he repeated over and over. The words began to blur with sobs.

The popping stopped. David's crying kept going, not stopping for at least five minutes.

Their mom said, "David, I know you are a good boy. Fighting at school for any reason is a mistake. You'll have a paddling any time it happens. Don't do it again."

"Yes, Mom," he sobbed.

"David---"

"Yes, Mom."

"I hope you understand. Did you know I had an uncle, Richard?"

"I know, but not much. He's dead isn't he?"

"Yes. He was a big young man, like you are a going to be a big man, 6'7" and 260 pounds. He got in a fight, hurt another man. When the police came he didn't want to go to jail. Fought them. Do you know what they did?"

"Made him go to jail?"

"No, David, they shot him, killed him. You have to understand, being big is a blessing, you can play ball, protect people, do all sorts of things better than other men or boys, just because you're big, but there's a price. You have to be in better control of yourself, and obey the rules more than ordinary boys. You could have hurt Billy. When you are older, if you yell at a policeman, or do something a little man might do and have it laughed off, they will kill you, and no one will blame them because of your size. Do you understand?"

"I'll be good, Mom."

"Yes, you will, and I'm going to hold you to a higher standard because I don't want to ever go to another funeral like Uncle Richard's---and I love you."

Glad it wasn't her, Ellen breathed another sigh of relief that day and the day the four-quart enema bag came home. She was laying on the floor her ear by the vent that day too. At first the vent was on blowing hot air in her ear and blocking part of the sound, and then it stopped.

David said, "Mom, how big's that bag?"

"Four-quarts."

"And the old one?" He asked.

"Two-quarts."

"Do I need four-quarts?"

Was there a lack of self confidence in his voice? David could be cocky, especially with Ellen, his little sister, not often with their mother, with their mother holding a four-quart enema bag in her hand.

David said, "Why?"

"The enemas I gave you yesterday weren't good enough, David. It takes more water to fill your colon, to get you well," their mother said.

Silence followed.

Ellen couldn't see, but she knew he was taking off his bathrobe and pajama bottoms. The bed creaked. Ellen heard that as he climbed on it and their mom sat down behind him, in her favorite position while giving enemas: behind her children with her hip against their lower backs. Her arm rested on David's hip, her hand holding the clamp after the nozzle was in, she supported him, loved him, made the enema more than a test of wills, made it a holding experience: the children holding the enema; she holding them. Hoisting the bag in the air with her other arm, she reminded Ellen of the Statue of Liberty with her enema bag torch, but their mom's torch, a red rubber bag, extinguished infections, fevers, and constipation; it didn't light up the night. Whatever huddle masses it promised freedom, were flushed. Mom's enemas weren't about liberty, but security, love and being a child in their mother's arms.

Mom said, "You all right, David?"

David said, "Yeah, all right."

Ellen listened another minute, maybe three.

Their mom said, "This bag's too heavy. I'm going to have to put a hook on the wall for it."

David said, "Maybe you need a lighter bag---like the old one."

"Nice try, David."

Ellen couldn't hear the click of the clamp being closed in her room, but she could hear the verbal effects of it being open.

David said, "Mom, I need to stop!"

"OK" Silence, some creaking of the bed, their mother was massaging his stomach.

The creaking of the bed stopped. Silence. "Mom!" He was full again.

A shorter wait before, "I've got to go!"

A little more enema, a beg, more enema, a beg, David was having trouble taking it.

Mom said, "David, you easily took the old bag, all of it, completely filling the colon to get the water into your system and flush out the bugs and get your body fighting back is important. You can take more than half of this bag, all I've given you so far. This time we need to work it and get everything in you that you can hold, then I'll know how big your colon is and how much water I need to use to treat you."

David said, "Mom, two-quarts is plenty, more than enough."

Mom said, "Breathe deep. Relax into it."

David was quiet. A minute passed. He groaned. More squeaking, Mom was massaging his stomach again.

Ellen timed it, looking at her wrist watch: 14 minutes. Their mom was still giving him the enema.

He kept saying, "Mom!" A periodic metronome steady with respiration, unsteady with tone. The pitch grew higher. His base voice, the one he was so proud of as he passed into being a teenager, was back to a childlike falsetto. He was taking an enema to remember.

At the end, he begged, "Please, Mom! I can't take any more!"

She said, "Were almost done, David. Only a cup or two, at most, is left in the bag. Breathe out and hold it out and your enema will be over."

A moment of silence, Ellen closed her eyes, imagined, could see the bag. It was going flat, the last little bulge on the bottom shrinking and folding up as suction collapsed the center and wrinkled the edges. His enema was in, all four quarts of it.

"OK, we're done," their mom said. "Now hold it for 15 minutes and you're done."

Mom left David, going down stairs to start dinner. Getting up, Ellen glanced at her wrist watch, got a book, laid it on her desk, started reading and waited to hear her mother on the stairs. She didn't come in 15 minutes. The toilet flushed twice before she came back. Ellen heard their mother's door open and close, dove for her spot by the vent.

David said, "That was an enema, Mom, a good enema."

"That's what a good enema means, David, as much as you can comfortably hold, an enema that fills and slightly stretches the whole colon. What you needed."

David was quiet.

Mom said, "David, aren't you glad I got the new bag?"

David said, "Yea, but don't tell anybody I said so."

"You're a good son."

David said, "Mom, if I need an enema, it might as well be a good one. I feel better."

Ellen got up, brushed her dress off and headed down stairs.

A few weeks later, having avoided telling her mother she was constipated, Ellen passed gas. Even if Mom had sinus problems, she couldn't miss that one.

She said, "Ellen, are you all right?"

"I'm OK, Mom," Ellen said. "It's---its fine, Mom."

Her mom said, "Look at me."

Ellen did. From three feet away her mother kept watching her face.

"You have that little crease."

"I don't have a crease, Mom!"

Ellen looked up trying to see the space between her own eyes.

"You have a headache."

"It's just a little one, Mom. I'll take an aspirin."

"You're constipated. You'll take an enema," Mom said. "How long have you been constipated?"

"A few days---four, I think."

"You'll take a few enemas then."

David was listening to the radio, or was he? He came in right at the end of their conversation during a commercial, got a glass of juice and went back in the living room to his program. Ellen watched his face; she didn't see that light in his eyes. He didn't hear anything. Ellen's first time with the big bag, she was glad no one else would ever know what was about to happen on her mother's bed.

Mom led her to the hall closet, got out the new enema bag and handed Ellen two towels, then went into the master bathroom. Ellen folded the spread back off the half of Mom's bed nearest the toilet. Mom didn't like the idea of salt stains from the tears of a paddling on her bed; enema stains were unthinkable. Ellen laid the towels out neatly, one on top of the other where her hips would go, then followed her mother into the bathroom.

Four tablespoons of baking soda in the bag, her mother was adjusting the water temperature in the tub faucet.

"Mom, I---" Ellen said, unzipping her skirt and taking off her panties, but her mother wasn't listening. Her mother was busy. The four quart bag was filling.

Her brother lounged comfortably on the couch in the living room listening to the radio. In her mother's bedroom, Ellen lay on her side on two towels.

Ellen was clenching her buttocks together, holding on as her mother held up the bag. Her colon stretched to take hold of the last few ounces of the good enema. She quivered.

"Mom, I've got to go!"

"Breathe deep, Ellen, you're doing fine. Only a little more."

Her legs quivering, her buttocks contracting, some cramping, she was constipated, hadn't gone for four days. She should have told her mother sooner. Enemas cause cramps when the constipation goes untreated too long, gets hard. If she had had an enema earlier, it wouldn't have cramped. She was headachy, had been a crab and needed the enema, wanted the enema, but at that second she only wanted to be rid of it, to have the surging, bulging mass of water that filled her rectum, and now the entire of her colon, pouring in the toilet.

Taking it, holding it, quivering, longing to let it go, Ellen was uncomfortable, embarrassed.

Two more rounds with the four-quart enema bag and her mother looked at the brown muddy water in the toilet.

"Looks like all the solids are out. Go ahead, put your clothes on," her mother said.

Standing by the toilet, naked from the waist down, Ellen was a teenager, embarrassed, eager to put her panties and skirt back on, eager to be a teenager again, not a baby begging to go potty.

Leaving the bathroom, her mother left her alone. Sliding her panties up she got one leg on and another surge hit. She ran for the toilet, more solids. If her mother were there would she give her another enema? Did she need one? Looking out the bathroom window she saw her mother catching the trolley at the end of the street. They wouldn't talk this time.

A wave of contentment, a good feeling, euphoria swept over her: a post enema high. Ellen felt good for the first time in days. She tingled; she breathed deeply; she felt good, a good radiating around her bare bottom into her abdomen and floating over her head.

She wanted to say, *Thanks, Mom.*

Her mother gone, the enema bag hung drying from the bathroom door, Ellen's panties still on the bedroom floor. She stood looking at the bag. Having enemas felt good, she enjoyed the feelings; she wanted to tell her Mom, to talk about it.

How could she talk about it? Enemas, bowel movements, nasty stuff, no one talked about enemas. Did other girls from school have enemas? If they did, they never said anything about it. Ellen never said anything about enemas. She looked at the bag, enjoyed the clarity, the relief, and walked into the hall.

Two hours taking, holding and releasing enemas in her mother's bedroom and her brother had left the couch. Amazing. Why was he standing in the hall?

He said, "Feel better, Sis?"

She didn't answer. *Where had he been?* "I thought you were listening to the radio, David!"

"I was. Jimmy Durante was singing."

Neurons spinning in her newly cleared brain, Ellen thought, *Wait a minute; he listened to things, yes, but on Saturday? He listened to music, but he didn't like Jimmy Durante. If Jimmy Durante was scheduled, he'd read, play ball, or do something else. They only got one radio station. He wouldn't listen to Jimmy if you paid him.*

He smiled.

Ellen said, "You've been reading in your room---since Mom and I came upstairs?"

He smiled.

Ellen's face burned red.

Ellen thought, *The pervert, the peeping tom, the listening tom. Why did he do that? Did he do that? He might have been reading. He has a book in his hand.*

They walked down the stairs, David following Ellen.

"I'm going over to George's, shoot some hoops," David said leaving her alone in the house.

Watching him round the corner, Ellen raced upstairs, turned the radio on beside her mother's bed on low, loud enough to hear it in the room, but not the hall. She slipped into David's room, lay by the heater vent. She could here every word, every note.

Ellen said, "I hated my brother. I should have hated my brother, shouldn't I?"

Veterans

My nurse came back in.

"It's been fifteen minutes, are you ready?"

"Yes!" I was up.

Glancing back, I saw the look of abandonment on Ellen's face. I thought, *No she shouldn't hate her brother, nor should she blame herself for hating him.*

"I'll be back. We'll talk."

When I came out of the toilet Ellen was sitting cross legged on her bed waiting for me.

Ellen said, "Do you feel better?"

I breathed in, a deep breath, one unblocked penetrating all the way through my cleared abdomen into my pelvis. Completely filled with cool, fresh air, light, floating, happy, the way you only feel after a complete bowel movement, I was euphoric.

I said, "Yes, and can I tell you a secret?"

"Sure," my sixteen-teen-year-old roommate said.

"Enemas feel good. I always feel good after an enema. Is that the way you feel about them?"

What was I saying, and why was I saying it to this kid. Yes, enemas feel good, but no one says that. We all lie, make like we hate them because it is a pooh pooh thing, something that is supposed to be disgusting, not talked about. But after that workout with the nurse and the huge release, I really did feel good, wanted to talk about it, to tell someone about it, wanted to see my mother smile down at me, say "you're a good girl" and tell someone I was a good girl.

I had taken a good enema, held it, got it in the toilet. A fundamental, elemental accomplishment, one basic to my humanity, to being toilet-trained, to being a four year-old girl again with my momma praising me. I wanted to talk, to listen, to hear words of encouragement, to encourage this girl, make her feel love, not hate, to help her be proud of herself for the elemental reason of her being Ellen.

She said, "I haven't been constipated since then. Well, maybe a little with my periods, but I didn't tell Momma. Do you think I should tell her?"

I said, "Do you want her to give you another good enema?"

Ellen looked down, she didn't answer.

After a long pause she said, "I didn't mind. The enemas made me feel better."

"Then tell your mother when you need one, I'm sure she will help you."

She said, "I guess I should."

She was blushing.

I said, "Why don't you then?"

"It's embarrassing, asking for an enema."

I said, "I was embarrassed, having that enema with you listening. I have always been embarrassed about enemas and would be embarrassed to ask for one."

Ellen said, "I'm sorry. I shouldn't have said so much. It's just---I wanted to talk about it after Momma gave me those enemas, to make it OK for me to ask. It didn't happen. Your---well, your having an enema---I'm sorry I talked too much."

"Now's your chance, Ellen, I'm here. We aren't going anywhere. If you want to talk about your feelings, I'll listen. As a matter of fact, if I am going to spend the next few hours taking enemas, I'd be glad to listen to you. OK?"

The nurse came in. "Are you ready for another enema?"

Twenty five minutes later, sitting on the toilet, the enema flowing out, I thought of my daughter. My daughter was three weeks younger than this girl. When was the last time we talked like Ellen and I were talking? Had we ever talked about something as intimate as an enema and how we feel about them? I'd never given her an enema. Shannon stayed with my mother one summer. My Mother gave enemas, but not like the nurse. Did she give Shannon enemas that summer? I never asked.

Holding the enema made it easier to be listening. I felt like listening, was learning, actually able to talk to a teenage girl. She was making sense, or was it the surging in my bowel, the intimacy of the enema that opened my mind to listen. Why couldn't my daughter talk to me like this? All Shannon and I did recently was argue. When she was crabby, we argued. I, the Mom, always told her what to do, or what not to do. If I listened to her, it was to judge her, not listening to her or letting her tell me her feelings.

Light stepping, I reentered our hospital room. Ellen was waiting for me.

I said, "I feel better, yet!"

I wanted to let her talk, share her feelings. We had been in the room together for four hours before my enemas, and not talked at all. Now we were confederates of the good enema, both knowing the surges and urges, veterans of the colonic wars, sharing war stories.

I said, "How to you feel, Ellen?"

"Nervous, I've never had surgery before." She showed me the mole on her back.

"You'll be fine, I'm sure," I said.

She looked at me, up and down: furtive glances again.

She said, "I'd rather be you, having some enemas, some tests, and going home."

"A good enema might relax you," I said.

She blushed.

I said, "Why don't you ask the nurse? I'd be less embarrassed if it was both of us having enemas, and it would relax you."

She turned red.

The nurse came in, said, "How are you doing?"

I said, "I'm fine---"

Ellen interrupted.

"Nurse, I've been uncomfortable all day. I think---I need to go to the bathroom."

The nurse said, "Do you want an enema?"

Ellen turned quickly, lying in her bed looking away from us, not saying anything.

The nurse said, "See if you can go. I'll come back in ten minutes and give you an enema if you can't."

Ellen, not looking at either of us, sprang from her bed and ran for the toilet.

The nurse said, "Poor kid, she's probably been constipated for days, wouldn't tell anybody. An enema will help her."

I smiled.

Twenty minutes later the nurse was giving Ellen her enema.

After Ellen, I had another good enema as Ellen empathized, even came over and pulled my blanket up to make me more comfortable while I was holding the last one.

"Thank you, Ellen," I said.

She said, "Thank you."

I smiled.

She said, "Thank you, I---I hadn't been able to go for three days, ever since the doctor scheduled me for surgery. I get like that. I get constipated if something bothers me."

I said, "Didn't they ask you about your BMs when you checked in?"

She blushed.

She said, "I told them I'd been having BMs."

"Why?"

"I don't know. If you hadn't told me to ask for an enema, I'd still have a headache. Thank You!"

We were new friends. She kept talking through our short stay, not just about enemas, about everything she wanted to talk to a grown person about, but was afraid to, afraid they wouldn't listen, afraid they would think she was silly, judge her. I was, and wasn't, a grown person to her. She knew I was old, had a daughter her age, but I was a person she heard having enemas, who had as hard a time holding on to them as she did. We were in the same class at school during the time we spent in the hospital. We were equals. Old legs quiver like young legs when getting good enemas.

Both of us left the next day.

When her mother came to pick her up after her surgery, I was back in the room after having had a Barium Enema. I missed the privacy, intimacy and friendship of the enemas in our room with Ellen, the nurse and I alone doing the enemas. In the X-ray room, it was very impersonal, people walking around the machine, the whirring of the machine. I felt like a slab of flesh on a table in our room with some of the nurses. In the x-ray room I was a slab of flesh hanging from a hook going down an assembly line. Two other patients waiting for Barium enemas after mine waited in the hall, and the one before me returned to the toilet spewing out more Barium and water while the X-ray technician filled me.

Ellen said, "I enjoyed talking to you. I never had a roommate before. It was sort of fun---Could I come to see you?"

I said, "I'd like that. I think Shannon would like to meet you too."

Ellen said to her mother, "Shannon's her daughter. She's three weeks younger than me."

Her mother said, "When? I can bring her over this weekend if you'd like?"

"Sure, we live at 315 Sycamore."

Her mother said, "Washington High."

I said, "Yes."

"Ellen's brother plays basketball for Jefferson." Then to Ellen she said, "You want to meet a girl from Washington. I thought you said the boys at Washington were all cads, or did after they beat Jefferson in the city championship."

Ellen said, "I'll meet her Mom. Not everyone from Washington is a cad, the girls are nice. It was just one boy that was nasty, called me short for a giraffe. Their coach made him apologize, too."

I looked at my new friend, shy about enemas; was she shy about her height? I wished this girl could play basketball, do sports. Her brother, a very tall boy, was a super star. Every coach wanted boys like him. But a girl? The tallest girl in her school, she was a freak. No one had to know about her feelings about enemas to know she was a freak. Looking up at her they could see she was strange, six-feet and one inch of strange. She needed a friend. Boy friends would be hard to find. So many of the age to date her killed in the war, the survivors having their pick of the field, most would opt for pretty little things on their arm. Likely, she would settle for a wounded hero, a man who needed her help, his arm around her shoulder helping him walk down the street.

Her mother would be crying when her husband came marching home in uniform, when it was over. She got a letter from Paul, was worried, scared, almost sick.

Somewhere in France, he survived Normandy, was moving toward Germany.

"He's with the army---a cook," Ellen's mother said. "I want him cooking at home. I want him home."

Visiting Ellen and seeing my closeness with her surprised my daughter, but at our house it changed over the first few minutes. Sitting at our table chatting, it wasn't just Ellen and I. It was the four of us. After a few sentences her Mom and I talked. Our daughters talked, or would have talked if we hadn't been in the room. They excused themselves and went to Shannon's room.

Before they left, my daughter said, "Can Ellen come to the sleep-over next weekend?"

My daughter and my new friend became friends. I became a mother, an old woman, too old for either of them to talk to as Ellen had talked to me in the hospital.

During the sleep-over there was one special moment. Ellen came in the kitchen away from the other girls. We were alone.

"Ellen, the time I had with you in the hospital meant a lot to me," I said.

"Me, too," she said. "Mom and I are closer. Sometimes we talk more now. Thank you. How about you and Shannon?"

"I'm still her Mom. I don't think I'll ever be anything else to her. I'm not sure I want to be."

"She's lucky you're her Mom, Mrs. Johnson."

We hugged for the first time and the last time. I missed my young friend, was glad my daughter had a new friend.

Kids, they looked to me for advice, to tell them what to do, and talked among themselves. When I came in the room chatter stopped; the Mom was there. When I left, it came back like turning on a light switch. I missed my new young friend, but her mother was nice. We talked.

Two days after the sleep-over, a lazy Tuesday afternoon, my daughter and I were alone in the house.

Shannon said, "Mom, I'm sorry I'm so bitchy. I feel like my period is starting. I can't go to the bathroom. Can you help me?"

I said, "I'm going to give you a good enema."

Shannon looked down, couldn't look at me, and smoothed her skirt over her hips. She trembled. I took her in my arms and hugged her, took her hand in mine, led her to the hall closet, got out the new four-quart enema bag, the one I bought the day before, and handed her two towels.

"Shannon, have you had an enema before?"

She said, "No!" fumbling to unzip her skirt.

~~~~*~~~~

Books by J G Knox

Love Thine Enemas and Heal Thyself
An Enema, A Birthday Spanking, A Love Story
For the Love of Amber
Marisa and the Enema Fetish

Books available through special order at book stores and online bookstores worldwide

Novellas by J G Knox

Momma's Tears, A Story of Love and Overcoming Grief

Other short stories by J G Knox

Mrs. Smith, the Boarding School Enemas
Caught and Spanked
Tall Dark and Handsome
Honey, I'm Home

Novellas and short stories available at Amazon kindle, e-book stores, or in pdf at http://www.e-lovestories.com

To be placed on the mailing list for new publications, to obtain order prices direct from the publisher to any location in the world (We offer a substantial discount on direct orders and bulk orders, usually 40-50% off book store price), or to share observations about this book, or other books we have written, please write:

Love Truth and Life Publishing
PO Box 65130
Vancouver, WA
98665
Telephone 360-690-0842

We reprint books with corrections periodically, and appreciate anything that will make future editions better. Those submitting corrections we use will be sent a new copy of the next edition.